Everybody
COURAGE

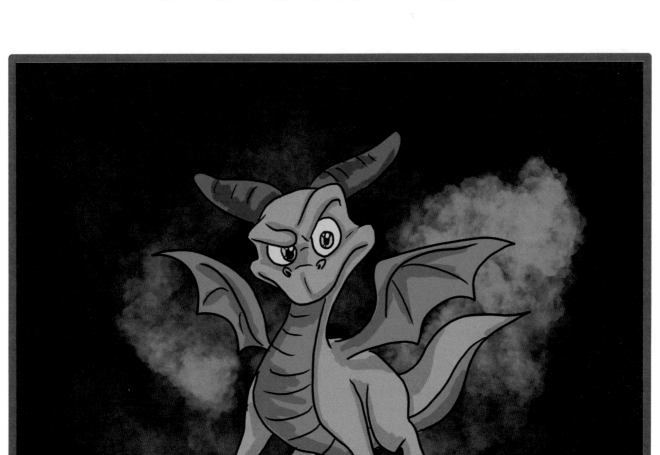

Co-Written & Illustrated by: Senetha Fuller
Co-Written by: J. Lavone Roberson

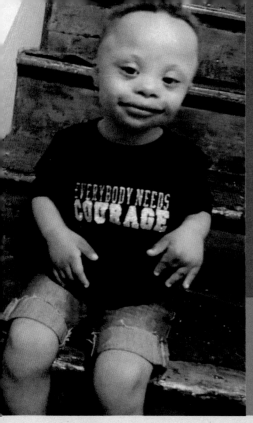

I dedicate this book to my everyday hero Courage who won his battle with cancer. To the ones continuing to fight - I'll take the weight if it will make you stronger.
#FightLikeCourage
-Senetha

SCAN ME

"Courage is not the absence of fear, it is the choice that something else is more important than being afraid." I dedicate this book to all of the children and caregivers who have been impacted by cancer. I hope this book reminds you that a little Courage goes a long way. -Lavone

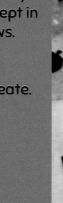
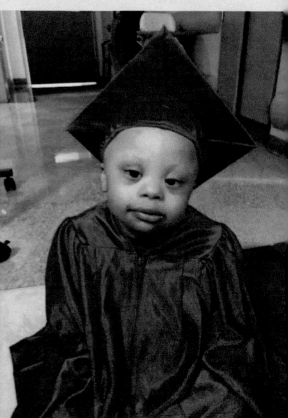

There once was a boy born mighty. Before he arrived his mother had a dream about a strong, happy, and brave boy. She named him *Courage*.

It was the only fitting name.

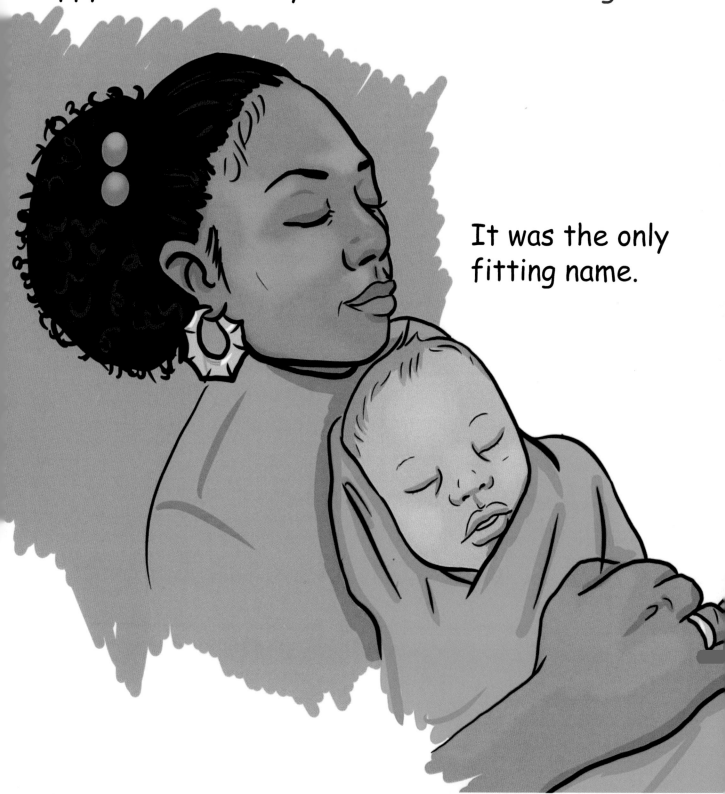

Courage lived in a small village. Everyone knew each other and everyone shared with one another.

Unfortunately, one season all of the villages children had become very ill. No one knew why.

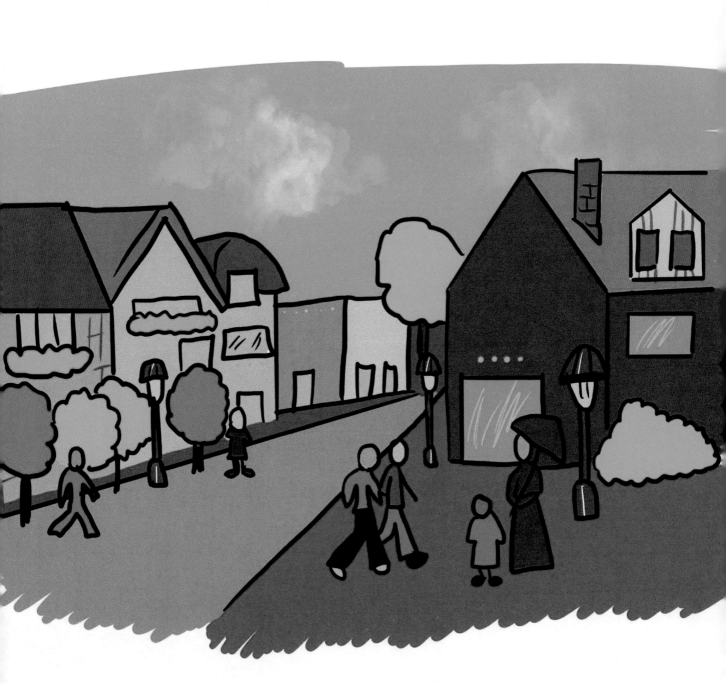

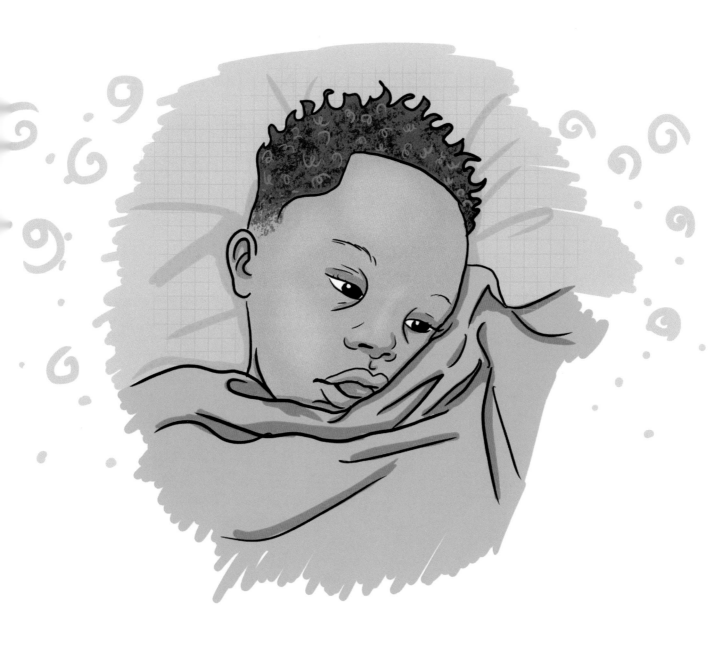

Courage was one of the children who got sick.
As months went by the other children got
better, but Courage did not.

Courage's mom and dad did everything they could to make him feel better but NOTHING worked!

They decided it was time to visit the doctor.

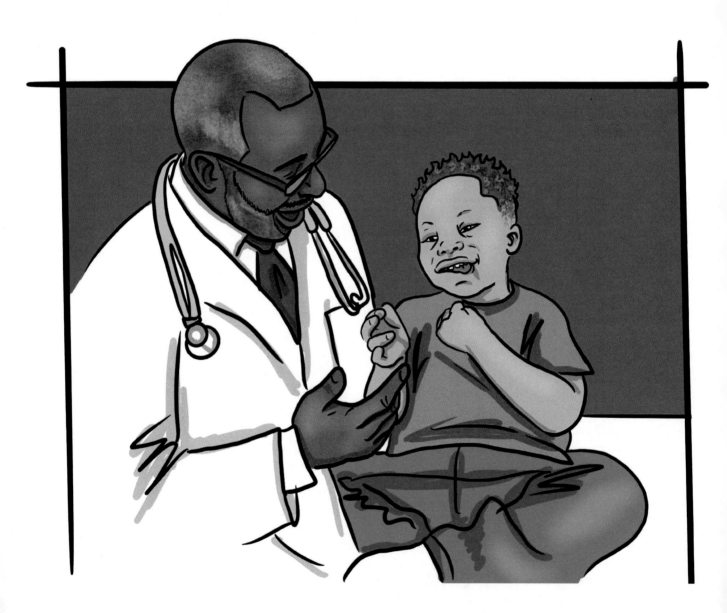

The doctor poked Courage with needles.
He checked his ears, his eyes, and checked his mouth.

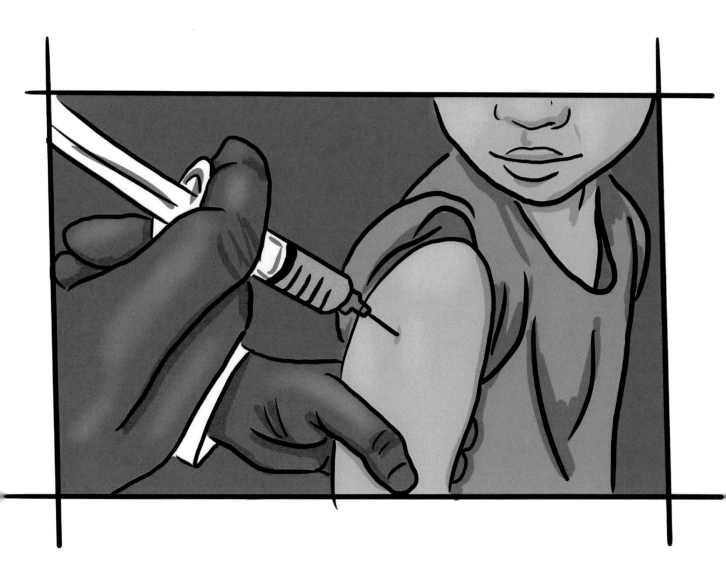

Courage did not cry or flinch.

"Courage is the right name for him. He is very brave!" The doctor said.

As Courage and his parents waited for the results his dad read him books about pirates, dragons, and adventures; Courage's favorite.

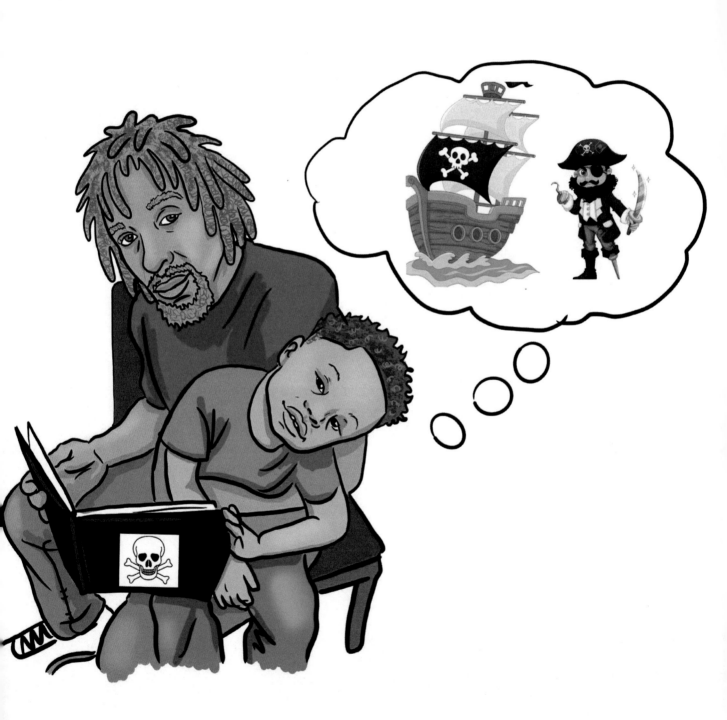

When the doctor came back he had some heart breaking news. "I am sorry to tell you this but it seems that Courage has something called Leukemia, cancer of the blood."

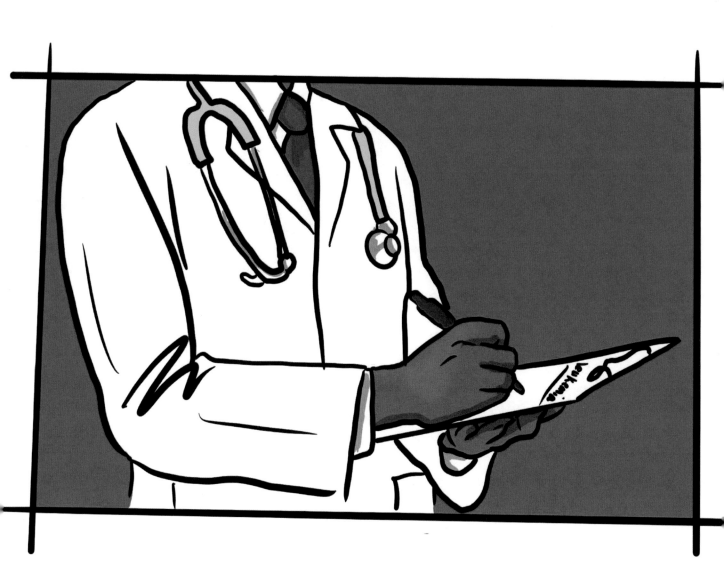

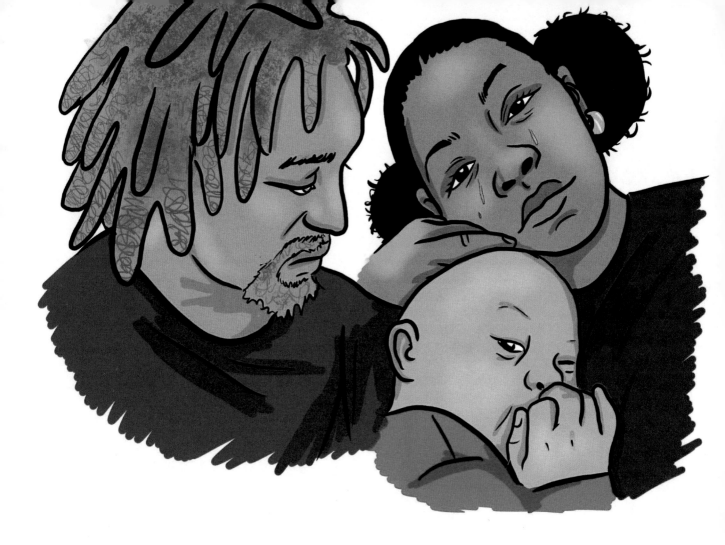

"Why?" His daddy asked.
"How?" His mommy cried.
They could not believe what they had heard.

Courage watched his parents cry. He was sad watching them worry. He knew he had to be brave for them. Everybody needs Courage, even Courage.

When his parents went to bed that night Courage lay awake in his bed.

He thought about the moments before his family heard about Leukemia.

He thought about the pirates and dragons that his father read to him about.

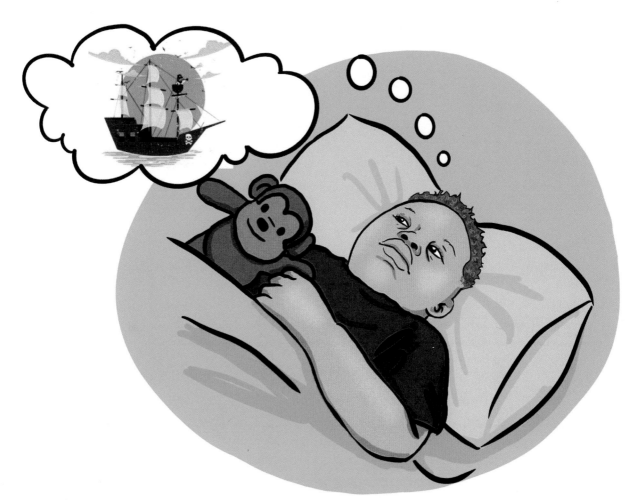

"I bet one of those evil dragons created cancer," he thought as he drifted to sleep.

The next thing he knew - he was in the middle of a forest!

"Where am I?"
"How did I get here?"
"I want to go home!"

There was only an echo.

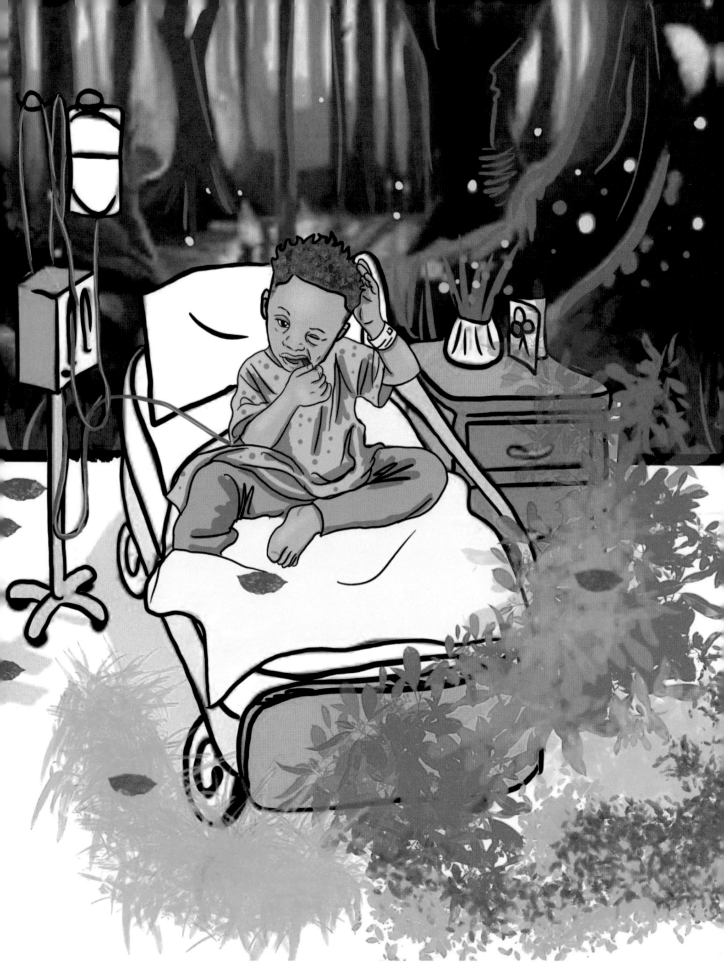

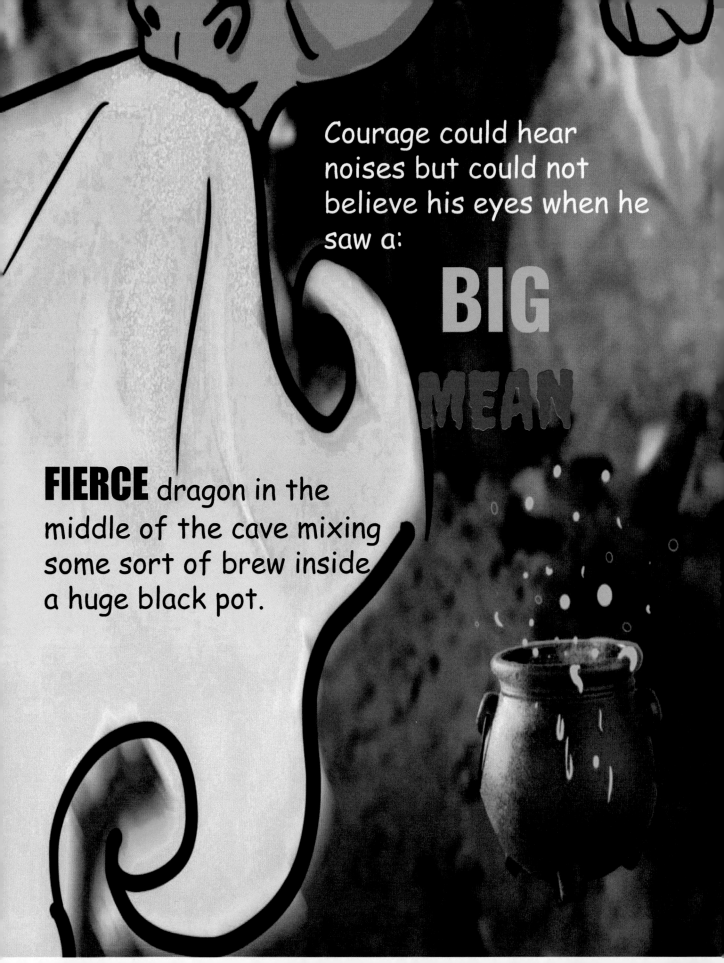

Courage could hear noises but could not believe his eyes when he saw a:

BIG MEAN

FIERCE dragon in the middle of the cave mixing some sort of brew inside a huge black pot.

The dragon was reciting a strange chant.

"Fiddle, swish, mix it quick, all of the children will be sick."
"Fiddle, swish, mix it quick, all of the children will be sick."

He mixed and mixed.

"I am the most powerful dragon!
I alone will gather all the world's children by
making them sick.
They will all work for meeeeee!"

Courage listened with sadness.

"Halt you BIG MEAN DRAGON! I am Courage and I will NOT let you hurt anyone else!" Courage yelled bravely.

"If all of the children are sick, all of the mommy's and daddy's will be sad.

The entire village would be ruined.

I will NOT let that happen!"

THE DRAGON STARED AT COURAGE.

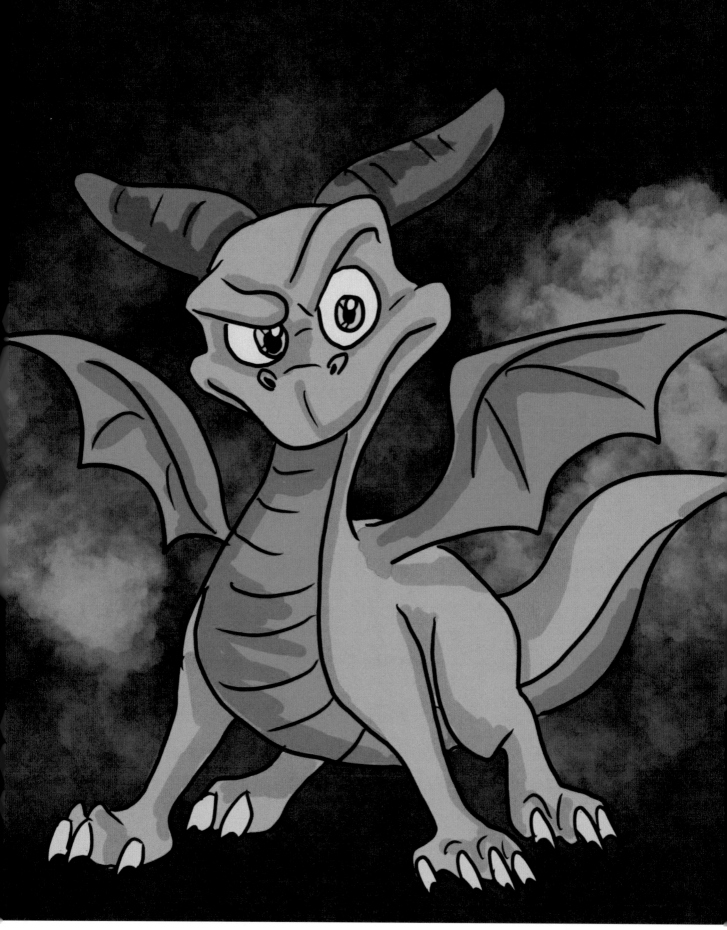

Courage picked up a stone and threw it at the dragon!

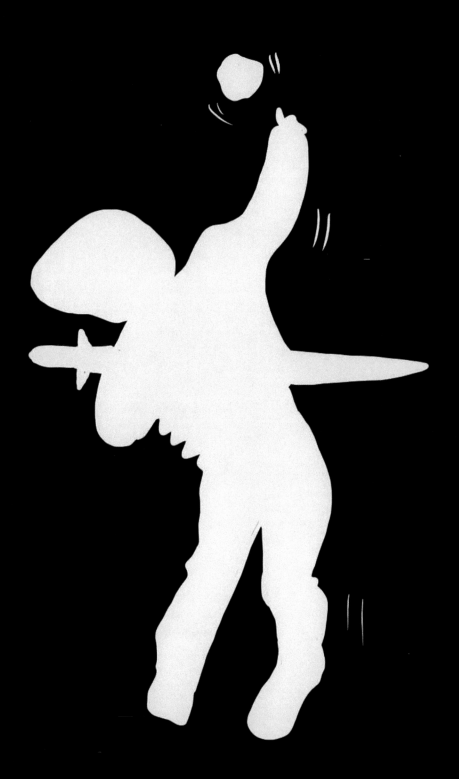

The dragon got closer to Courage and laughed.

MUA HAHAHAHA
"Look at you!
You're too small and weak to defeat me!
I am a big and powerful dragon
with a nose that has fire.
I will crush you with
one swipe of my tail!
It'll happen so fast
no one will hear you wail.
I have already mixed
my Leukemia brew and there is
nothing –
nothing –
nothing
you can do!"

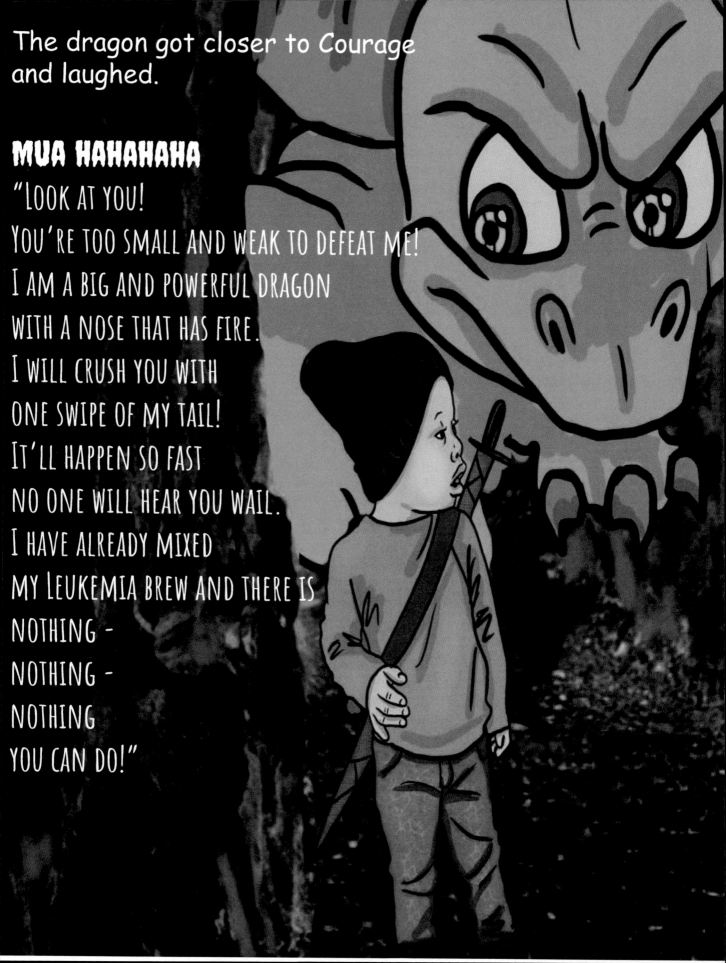

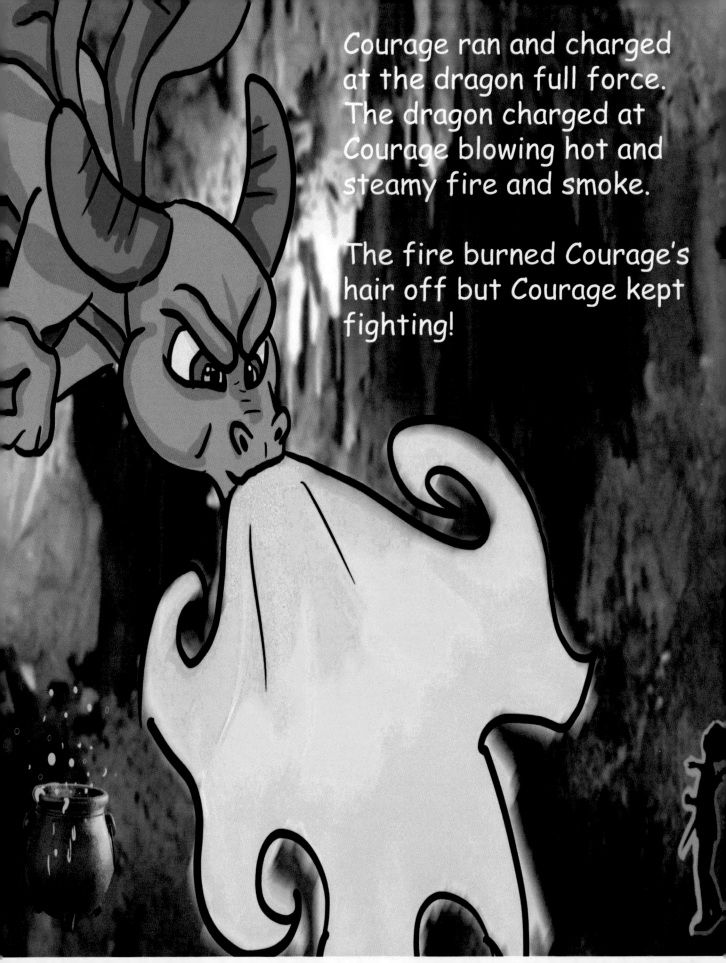

Courage ran and charged at the dragon full force. The dragon charged at Courage blowing hot and steamy fire and smoke.

The fire burned Courage's hair off but Courage kept fighting!

Courage ran in between the dragons feet.

Courage **jumped**. He *flipped*.

The dragon was big and strong.

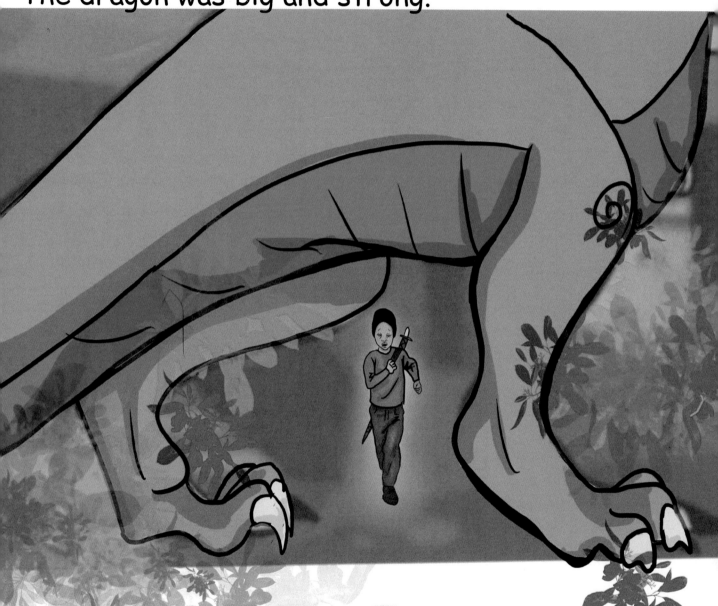

Courage started to worry that the dragon was going to catch him and eat him but **Courage kept fighting.**

Courage tickled him.
He spun around making the dragon fall on his back in a crash!

BOOM!

"HELP ME!
I HAVE FALLEN DOWN.
YOU BETTER GET ME
OFF THE GROUND!"

The mean dragon yelped!

I will help you only if you tell me what to add to this potion to make it help the children feel better.

"I CAN'T DO THAT!" THE DRAGON SAID.

Courage jumped on the pot with the brew and scooped some out to pour on the dragon!

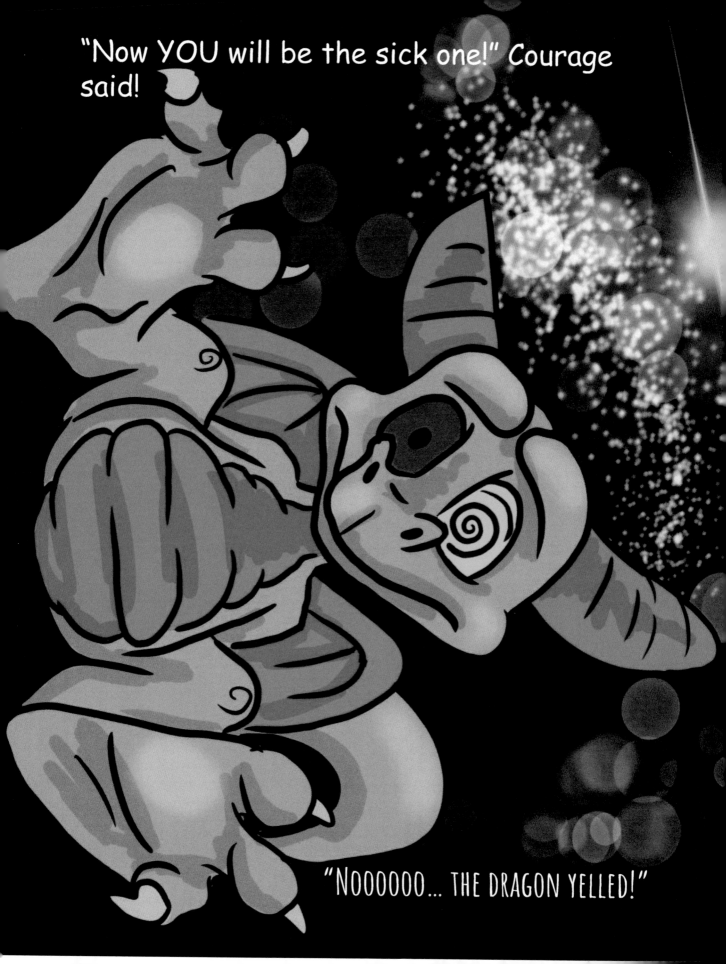

"Fine! I'll tell you!" He was trying to roll over.

"You are the secret ingredient Courage! I knew you'd come but never thought you'd defeat me. Hug the cauldron, give it a shake... and all of the sickness will go away."

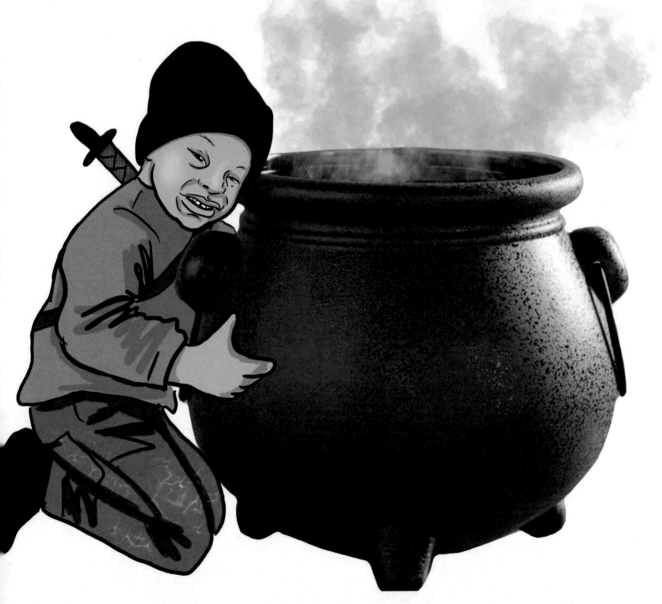

Courage hugged the cauldron and gave it a shake.

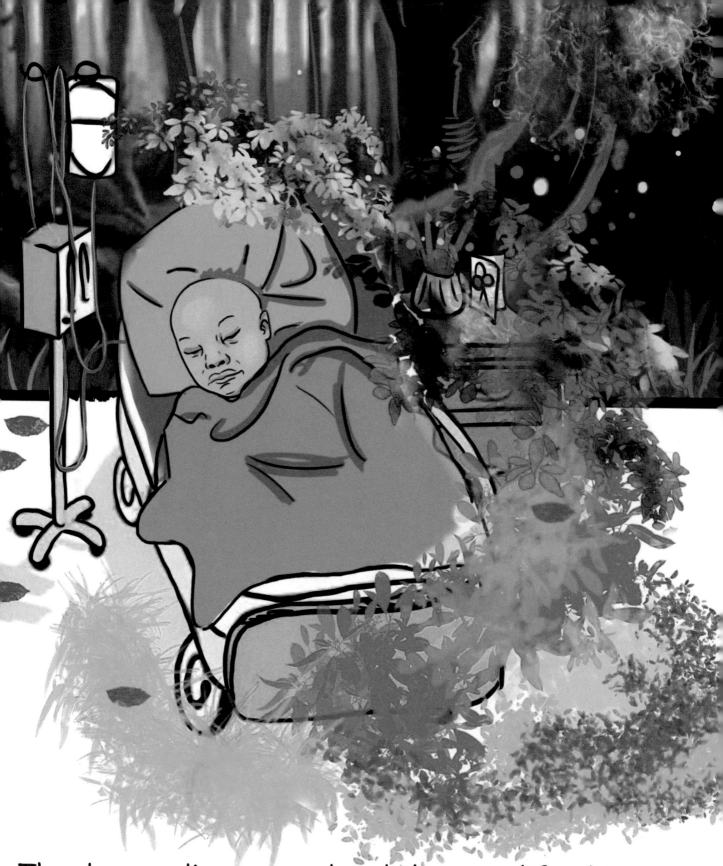

The dragon disappeared and the cave lifted into the air.

"Courage" wake up his mom said.
It's time to put on your cap and gown.
We are leaving the hospital. Somehow you beat
cancer, and you don't have Leukemia anymore.

You did it Courage!

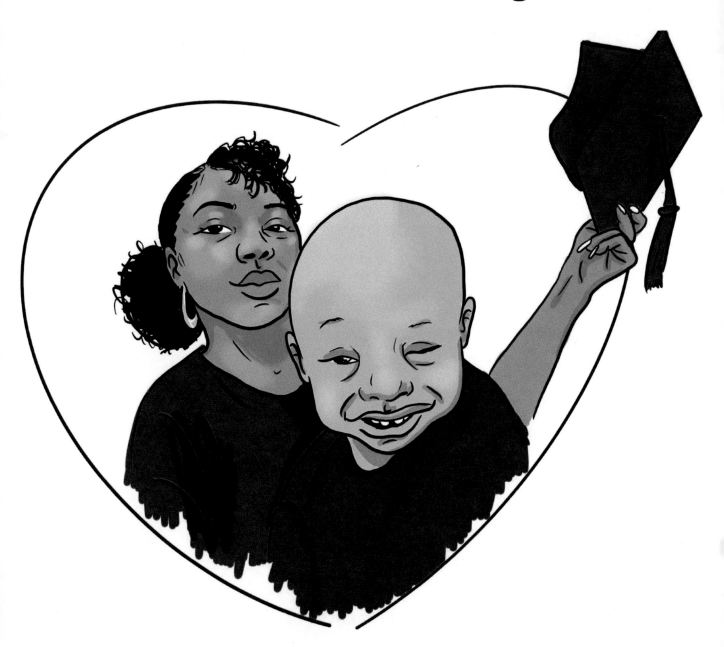

Brave young Courage cured his sickness.

The mayor handed
Courage a reward and
from then on was
labeled *The Bravest Boy
in the World.* Courage
the GREAT!

"You know,
**everybody needs a
little Courage.**" The
mayor said.

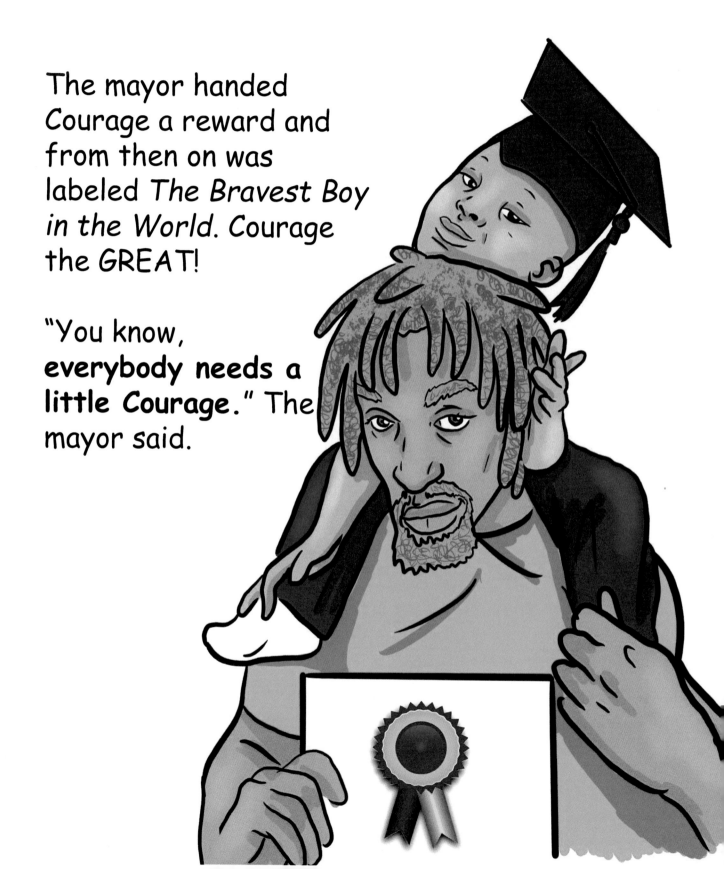

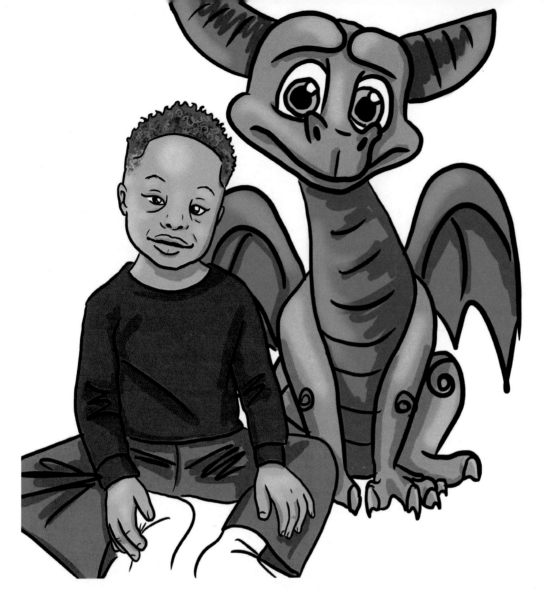

Courage never told anyone about that day with the dragon but whenever he sees someone in need - he still shares a hug and a shake to help them.

It may not cure all of the sicknesses in the world but he hopes to remind everyone that if you ever have to face a dragon ... all you need is a little Courage.

The Story of Courage Sabir

As told by his Mom Senetha Fuller

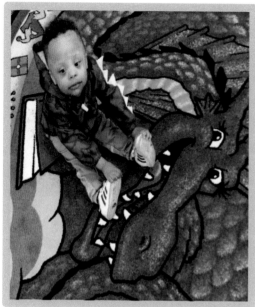

Courage Sabir was born on May 16, 2017. He was diagnosed with leukemia in April 2018. Before being diagnosed he had cold-like symptoms on and off, it seemed to last longer than it should. He would play, laugh, and crawl normally. At his routine doctor visit his doctor ran blood tests twice, which seemed odd.

The doctor eventually came in the room and told us that Courage had leukemia. I cried for what seemed like an eternity. Courage embraced his dad when the doctor told us we would not be going home. Courage started chemotherapy that day. He lived in the Philadelphia Children's Hospital for five months until he graduated from chemotherapy and we went home. Courage has been cancer free for 3 years.

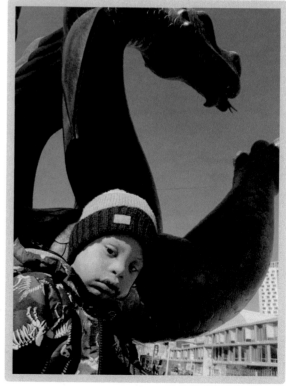

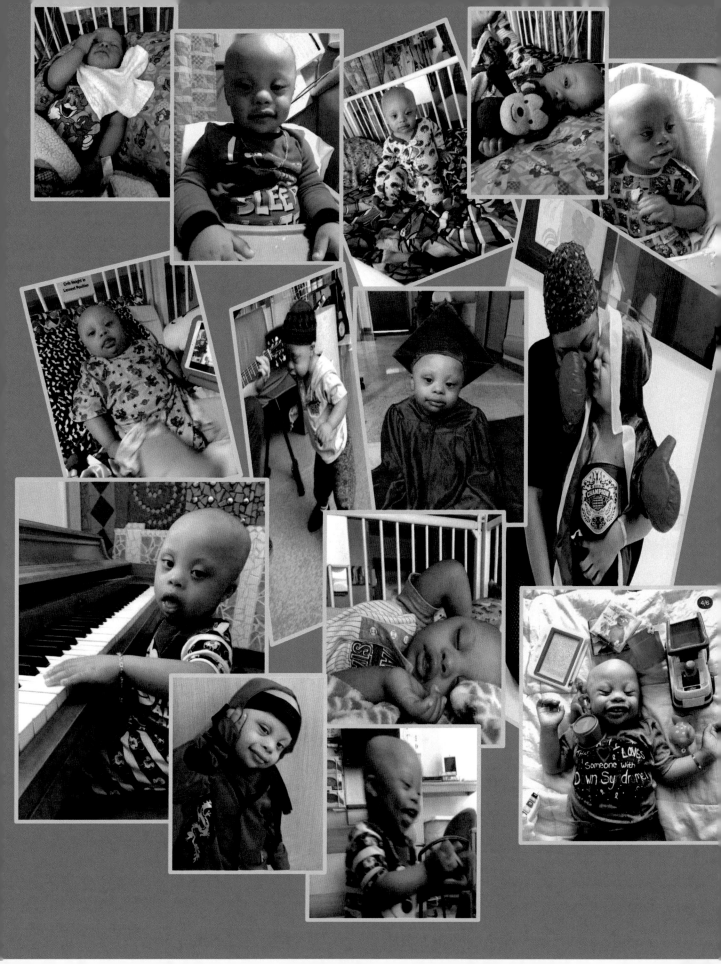

cour·age

/ˈkərij/ *(noun)*

- The ability to do something despite being afraid.
- Strength in the face of fear, pain, or grief.

Synonyms: bravery, heroism, fearlessness

When have you shown courage?

_____

_____

_____

What are you afraid of?

_____

_____

How could you show courage if you were ever faced with your fear?

_____

_____

_____

Author + Illustrator

Senetha Fuller resides in Philadelphia, PA. She specializes in "urban art" and creates custom art using different mediums. It has always been her passion to inspire through her art, and to create a book about her son Courage. @Red_Panda_Artz

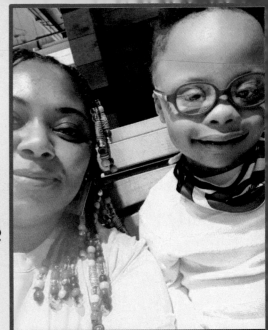

Scan here to read our other books.

SCAN ME

Jacquelyn "Lavone" Roberson – *Educator *Philanthropist *Author* is from Norwalk, CT. She is an educator and two time cancer survivor. She writes about Nia, a fictional character who helps people learn purpose. Lavone is The CEO and Founder of The Now I Am Nia Foundation, Inc, where she serves communities in need through various philanthropic projects. Lavone is an alumni of Hampton University and a member of Delta Sigma Theta Sorority, Incorporated. When she was a teacher she was selected with 5 of her colleagues to be the Nation's First Quad–D Lab Classroom. When she is not writing, teaching, or working in the community she enjoys traveling and spending time with her 6 god children. To learn more, donate, or book for speaking engagements please visit **www.NowIAmNia.org** and follow us **@NowIAmNia**.

Made in the USA
Middletown, DE
27 March 2022

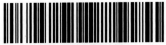